THE ULTIMATE PLANT BASED DIET COOKBOOK

50 Flexible plant based recipes for beginners and advanced to Lose weight and reset metabolism. Eat like a pro and cook easy and flavourful recipes even if you are busy

Ursa Males

TABLE OF CONTENTS

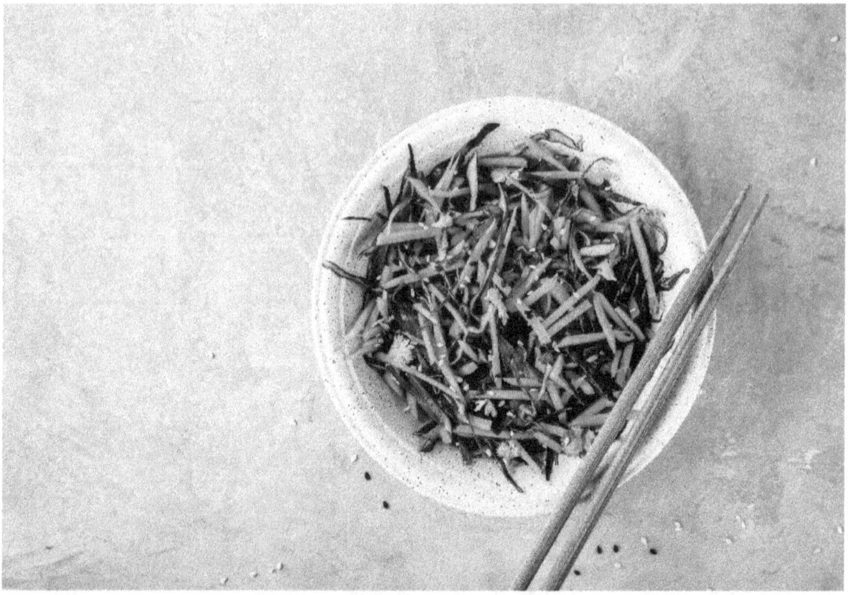

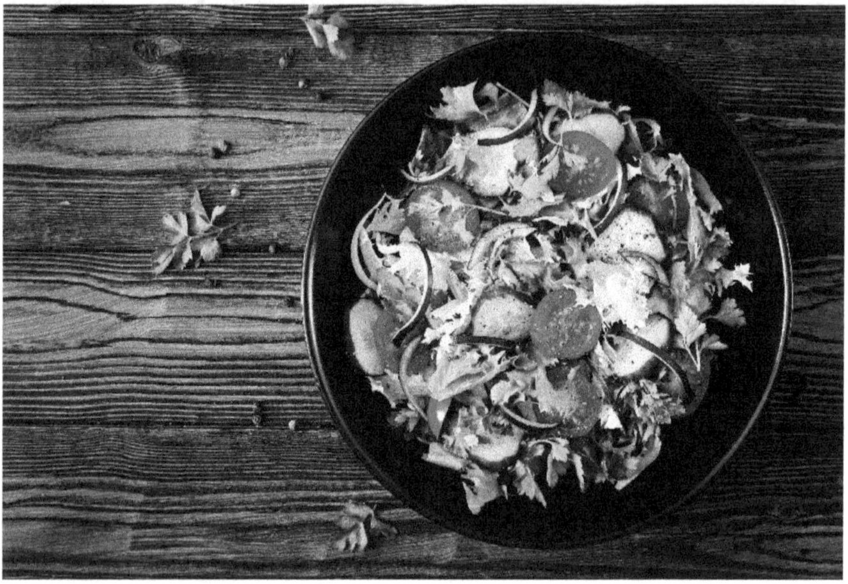

BREAKFAST

1. Granola Cereal

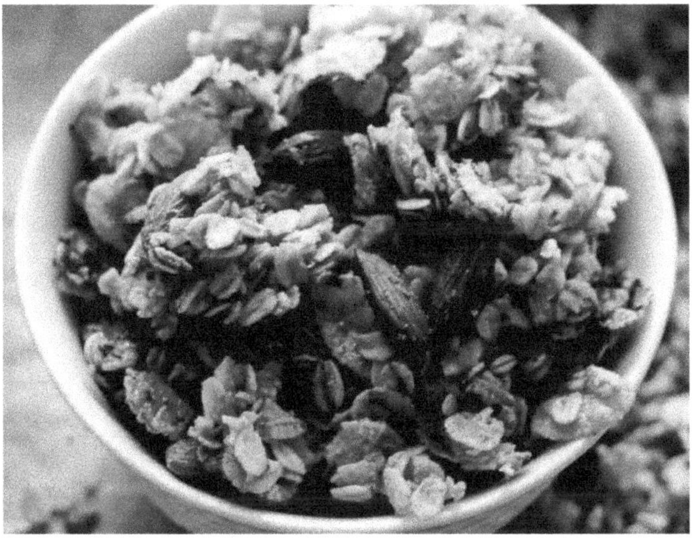

Preparation time: 15 minutes

Cooking time: 40 minutes

Servings: 10

Ingredients:

- 3 cups old-fashioned rolled oats
- 1/2 cup pecans, coarsely chopped
- 3/4 cup unsweetened shredded coconut
- 1/4 cup coconut sugar/brown sugar
- 1/2 teaspoon cinnamon

- 3/4 teaspoon sea salt
- 3/4 cup maple syrup
- 1 teaspoon vanilla extract
- 1 cup raisins

Directions:

1. Preheat oven to 300°F. Line 2 baking sheets with parchment paper. Combine the oats, pecans, coconut, sugar, cinnamon, and salt in a large bowl.
2. Combine maple syrup plus vanilla extract in a separate bowl. Combine both mixtures and evenly spread onto baking sheets.
3. Cook within 35 to 40 minutes until golden brown, stirring every 15 minutes to achieve an even color.
4. Remove from oven and let cool. Transfer into a large bowl. Add raisins and mix until well combined. Store in an airtight container.

Nutrition: Calories 280Fat 8g Carbohydrate 51g Protein 4g

2. Banana Pancakes

Preparation time: 15 minutes

Cooking time: 20 minutes

Servings: 10

Ingredients:

- 1 cup whole wheat flour
- 1 teaspoon baking powder
- 1/2 teaspoon cinnamon
- 1/4 teaspoon sea salt
- 1 large ripe banana
- 1 cup almond milk
- 1/4 cup unsweetened applesauce
- 1/2 teaspoon apple cider vinegar
- 1 teaspoon vanilla extract

Directions:

1. Combine all dry fixings in a medium-size bowl. Mash banana in a separate bowl. Combine wet ingredients with the mashed banana.
2. Mix the dry fixings with the wet fixings until well combined. Heat a nonstick pan on medium. Put a spoonful of the batter onto the pan and cook until bubbles begin to form.

3. Flip pancake and cook until golden color appears. Repeat until all the batter is gone. Drizzle with maple syrup and serve.

Nutrition: Calories 67 Fat 1g Carbohydrate 14g Protein 3g

3. Berry Buckwheat Breakfast Bake

Preparation time: 15 minutes

Cooking time: 30 minutes

Servings: 6

Ingredients:

- 1 cup buckwheat flour
- 2 tablespoons flax meal
- 1/2 teaspoon cinnamon
- 1/2 teaspoon baking soda
- 1/4 teaspoon sea salt
- 1/2 cup unsweetened almond milk
- 1/2 cup maple syrup
- 1 teaspoon vanilla extract
- 1 ripe banana
- 1 cup mixed berries

Directions:

1. Preheat oven to 350°F. Prepare a 9x9 baking dish lined using parchment paper. Combine the dry ingredients in a large bowl.
2. In a separate bowl, mix the almond milk, maple syrup, and vanilla extract. Mix the liquid with the dry ingredients.

3. Mash up the banana and stir into the mixture. Mix in the berries. Pour mixture into baking dish. Bake for approximately 30 minutes. Top with fresh fruit or maple syrup.

Nutrition: Calories 221Fat 2g Carbohydrate 49g Protein 5g

4. <u>Hash Brown Cakes</u>

Preparation time: 15 minutes

Cooking time: 10 minutes

Servings: 4

Ingredients:

- 2 potatoes, peeled and grated
- 1/2 small onion, diced
- 1/4 cup whole wheat flour
- 1 tablespoon nutritional yeast
- 1/2 teaspoon sea salt
- Black pepper to taste

Directions:

1. Peel and coarsely shred potatoes using a grater or in a food processor.
2. Rinse with cold water in your colander, then drain well and then pat dry with paper towels.
3. Place potatoes in a large bowl. Stir in the onions, flour, nutritional yeast, salt, and pepper. Mix well—Preheat a large nonstick skillet over medium heat.
4. For each cake, scoop 1/4 of the potato mixture onto the skillet. Press down the potato batter with a spatula to flatten evenly—Cook within 5 minutes.

5. Using a wide spatula, carefully turn potato cakes. Cook again within 3 to 5 minutes more or until golden brown.

Nutrition: Calories 110Fat 0gCarbohydrate 24gProtein 4g

5. Biscuits with Mushroom Gravy

Preparation time: 45 minutes

Cooking time: 28 minutes

Servings: 16 biscuits

Ingredients:

Biscuits:

- 2 cups whole wheat pastry flour
- 2 teaspoons baking powder
- 2 teaspoons baking soda
- 3/4 teaspoon sea salt
- 1 cup unsweetened almond milk
- 1 tablespoon lemon juice
- 1/2 cup cashew cream (1/2 cup water blended with 1/2 cup-soaked raw cashews)

Gravy:

- 3 tablespoons water for sautéing vegetables
- 1/2 cup onion, finely chopped
- 1 clove garlic, minced
- 2 cups cremini mushrooms, chopped
- 2 cups low-sodium vegetable broth
- 1 teaspoon of sea salt
- 1/2 teaspoon black pepper

- 1/4 cup unsweetened almond milk
- 1/4 cup whole wheat flour

Directions:

1. Preheat oven to 425°F. Line a baking sheet with parchment paper. For the biscuits, mix the dry ingredients.
2. Mix the almond milk, lemon juice, and cashew cream in a separate bowl. Combine both dry and wet ingredients.
3. Form into flat circles of dough and place on the baking sheet—Bake for 7 to 8 minutes.
4. For the gravy, water sauté chopped onions and garlic until golden. Put the mushrooms, then cook within a few more minutes.
5. Put in the vegetable broth, salt, plus pepper. Add in the almond milk. Whisk in the flour and keep stirring over low heat until the gravy thickens for approximately 15 to 20 minutes.

Nutrition: Calories 116Fat 4g Carbohydrate 17g Protein 5g

6. Breakfast Potato Casserole

Preparation time: 15 minutes

Cooking time: 1 hour & 10 minutes

Servings: 10

Ingredients:

Sauce:

- 1/2 cup unsweetened almond milk
- 1 yellow bell pepper, chopped
- 1/4 cup raw cashews
- 1/2 cup nutritional yeast
- 1/2 teaspoon spicy brown mustard
- 1/2 teaspoon paprika
- 1/2 teaspoon turmeric
- 1 1/2 teaspoons sea salt
- 1/4 teaspoon black pepper
- Dash of cayenne pepper

Casserole:

- 3 tablespoons water for sautéing vegetables
- 1 small yellow onion, diced
- 1 small red bell pepper, diced
- 1 small orange bell pepper, diced
- 7 gold potatoes, chopped into small cubes

Directions:

1. Preheat oven to 350°F. Set aside a 9x13 casserole dish. Place all sauce ingredients into a blender. Blend at high speed until smooth. Set aside.
2. Heat-up a large nonstick skillet over medium-high heat. Sauté onion until softened. Stir in bell peppers and continue to sauté until the vegetables become tender. Add in the potatoes.
3. Allow mixture to heat through for a couple of minutes. Add the blended sauce mixture and stir to combine evenly.
4. Transfer potato and vegetable mixture to the casserole dish. Cover with foil—Bake for 45 to 50 minutes.
5. Uncover and continue to bake for an additional 15 to 20 minutes or until the top is golden brown. Remove from oven and serve.

Nutrition: Calories 173Fat 3gCarbohydrate 30gProtein 8g

7. Southwestern Tofu Scramble

Preparation time: 15 minutes

Cooking time: 10 minutes

Servings: 4

Ingredients:

- 14 ounces extra-firm tofu
- 1/4 cup low-sodium vegetable broth
- 1 red onion, diced
- 1 red bell pepper, thinly sliced
- 1/2 cup cremini mushrooms, chopped
- 1/4 cup nutritional yeast
- 1 teaspoon garlic powder
- 1 teaspoon cumin powder
- 1/2 teaspoon smoked paprika
- 1/2 teaspoon chili powder
- 1/2 teaspoon crushed red pepper
- 1/4 teaspoon turmeric
- 3/4 teaspoon sea salt
- Black pepper to taste
- Optional toppings: salsa, cilantro, hot sauce

Directions:

1. Pat tofu dry and absorb any excess liquid with a paper towel or clean cloth. Set aside. Heat a large skillet over medium heat.
2. Sauté the onions, red bell pepper, and mushrooms in the vegetable broth for approximately 5 minutes.
3. Take the tofu and crumble it into bite-sized pieces into the skillet. Add in the nutritional yeast and seasonings and cook for another 5 to 7 minutes until tofu is slightly browned.
4. Top with salsa, cilantro, or hot sauce. Serve immediately with breakfast potatoes, toast, or fruit.

Nutrition: Calories 116 Fat 2g Carbohydrate 11g Protein 14g

8. Gorgeous Green Smoothie

Preparation time: 5 minutes

Cooking time: 0 minutes

Servings: 2

Ingredients:

- ¼ cup nut or seed butter
- 2 frozen bananas, peeled
- 4 cups tightly packed shredded leafy greens
- 2 tablespoons chia seeds

Directions:

1. Combine all the fixings in a blender and add 3 cups of water. Purée for 30 seconds to 1 minute, until most of the green flecks have disappeared and the texture is smooth and creamy.

Nutrition: Calories: 380 Fat: 22g Protein: 12g Carbs: 41g

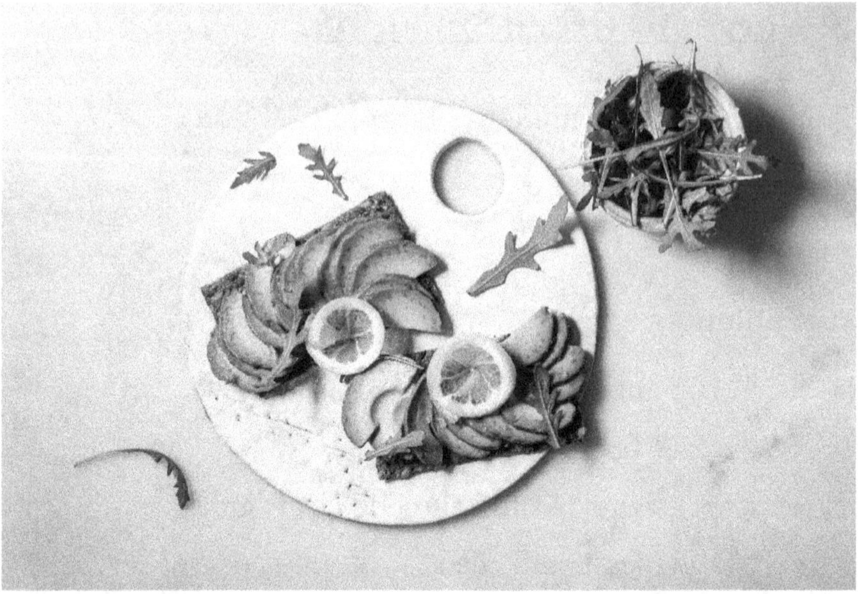

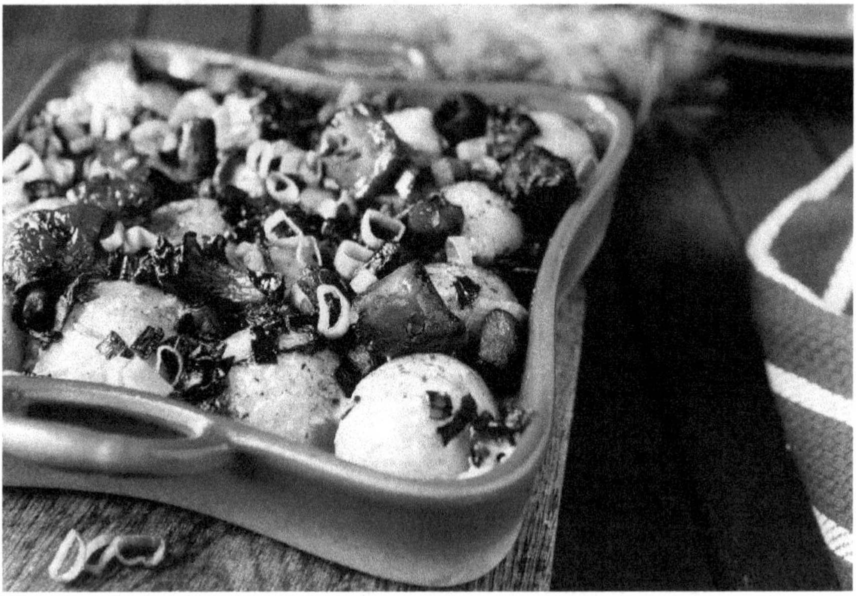

LUNCH

9. Pumpkin and Brussels Sprouts Mix

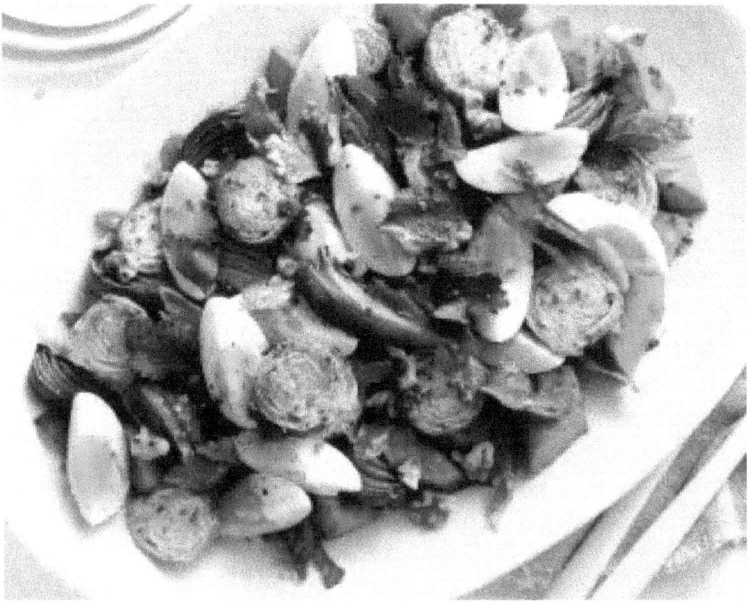

Preparation time: 15 minutes

Cooking time: 35-40 minutes

Servings: 8

Ingredients:

- 1 lb. Brussels sprouts, halved
- 1 pumpkin, peeled, cubed
- 4 garlic cloves, sliced
- 2 tablespoons fresh parsley, chopped

- 2 tablespoons balsamic vinegar
- 1/3 cup olive oil
- Salt, pepper, to taste

Directions:

1. Warm oven to 400 degrees F. Prepare a baking dish and coat with cooking spray. Mix sprouts, pumpkin and garlic in a bowl. Add oil and toss well to coat the vegetables.
2. Transfer to the baking dish and cook for 35-40 minutes. Stir once halfway. Serve topped with parsley.

Nutrition: Calories 152Fat 9 g Carbohydrate 17 g Protein 4 g

10. Almond and Tomato Salad

Preparation time: 15 minutes

Cooking time: 10 minutes

Servings: 4

Ingredients:

- 1 cup arugula/ rocket
- 7 oz fresh tomatoes, sliced or chopped
- 2 teaspoons olive oil
- 2 cups kale
- 1/2 cup almonds

Directions:

1. Put oil into your pan and heat it on a medium heat. Add tomatoes into the pan and fry for about 10 minutes. Once cooked, allow it to cool. Combine all salad ingredients in a bowl and serve.

Nutrition: Calories 355Fat 19.1 g Carbohydrate 8.3 g Protein 33 g

11. Strawberry Spinach Salad

Preparation time: 15 minutes

Cooking time: 0 minutes

Servings: 4

Ingredients:

- 5 cups baby spinach
- 2 cups strawberries, sliced
- 2 tablespoons lemon juice
- 1/2 teaspoon Dijon mustard
- 1/4 cup olive oil
- 3/4 cup toasted almonds, chopped
- 1/4 red onion, sliced
- Salt, pepper, to taste

Directions:

1. Take a large bowl and mix Dijon mustard with lemon juice in it, and slowly add olive oil and combine. Season the mixture with black pepper and salt.
2. Now, mix strawberries, half cup of almonds, and sliced onion in a bowl. Pour the dressing on top and toss to combine.

3. Serve the salad topped with almonds and vegan cheese.

Nutrition: Calories 116Fat 3 g Carbs 13 g Protein 6 g

12. Apple Spinach Salad

Preparation time: 15 minutes

Cooking time: 0 minutes

Servings: 4

Ingredients:

- 5 ounces fresh spinach
- 1/4 red onion, sliced
- 1 apple, sliced
- 1/4 cup sliced toasted almonds

For the Dressing:

- 3 tablespoons red wine vinegar
- 1/3 cup olive oil
- 1 minced garlic clove
- 2 teaspoons Dijon mustard
- Salt, pepper, to taste

Directions:

1. Combine red wine vinegar, olive oil, garlic, and Dijon mustard in a bowl. Season with black pepper and salt.
2. In a separate bowl mix fresh spinach, apple, onion, toasted almonds. Pour the dressing on top and toss to combine.
3. Serve

Nutrition: Calories 232Fat 20.8 g Carbs 10 g Protein 3 g

13. <u>Kale Power Salad</u>

Preparation time: 15 minutes

Cooking time: 40 minutes

Servings: 2

Ingredients:

- 1 bunch kale, ribs removed and chopped
- 1/2 cup quinoa
- 1 tablespoon olive oil
- 1/2 lime, juiced
- ½ teaspoon salt
- 1 tablespoon olive oil
- 1 red rose potato, cut into small cubes
- 1 teaspoon ground cumin
- 3/4 teaspoons salt
- 1/2 teaspoon smoked paprika
- 1 lime, juiced
- 1 avocado, sliced into long strips
- 1 tablespoon olive oil
- 1 tablespoon cilantro leaves
- 1 jalapeno, deseeded, membranes removed and chopped
- salt
- ¼ cup pepitas

Directions:

1. Rinse quinoa in a running water for 2 minutes. Mix 2 cups water and rinsed quinoa in a pot, reduce heat to simmer and cook for 15 minutes.
2. Remove quinoa from heat and let rest, covered, for 5 minutes. Uncover pot, drain excess water and fluff quinoa with a fork. Let cool.
3. Warm-up olive oil in a pan over medium heat. Add chopped red rose potatoes and toss. Add smoked paprika, cumin and salt. Mix to combine.
4. Add ¼ cup water once pan is sizzling. Cover the pan then adjust heat to low. Cook for 10 minutes, stirring occasionally. Uncover pan, raise heat to medium and cook for 7 minutes. Set aside to cool.
5. Transfer kale to a bowl and add salt to it and massage with hands. Scrunch handfuls of kale in your hands. Repeat until kale is darker in color.
6. Mix 2 tablespoons olive oil, ½ teaspoon salt and 1 lime juice in a bowl. Add over the kale and toss to coat.
7. Add 2 avocados, 2 lime juices, 2 tablespoons olive oil, jalapeno, cilantro leaves and salt in a blender. Blend well and season the avocado sauce.
8. Toast pepitas in a skillet over medium low heat for 5 minutes, stirring frequently. Add quinoa to the kale bowl and toss to combine well.

9. Divide kale and quinoa mixture into 4 bowls. Top with red rose potatoes, avocado sauce, and pepitas. Enjoy!

Nutrition: Calories 250Fat 11 g Carbs 25 g Protein 9 g

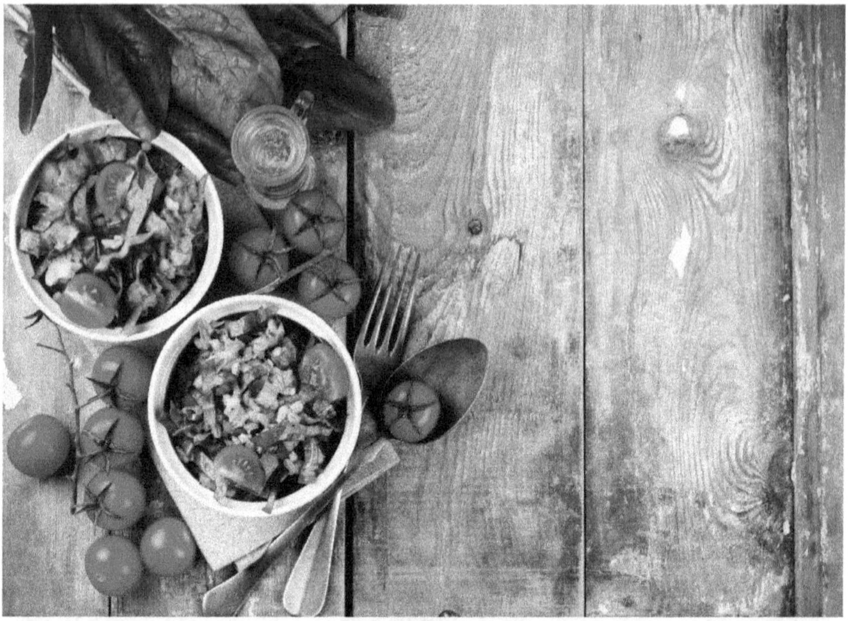

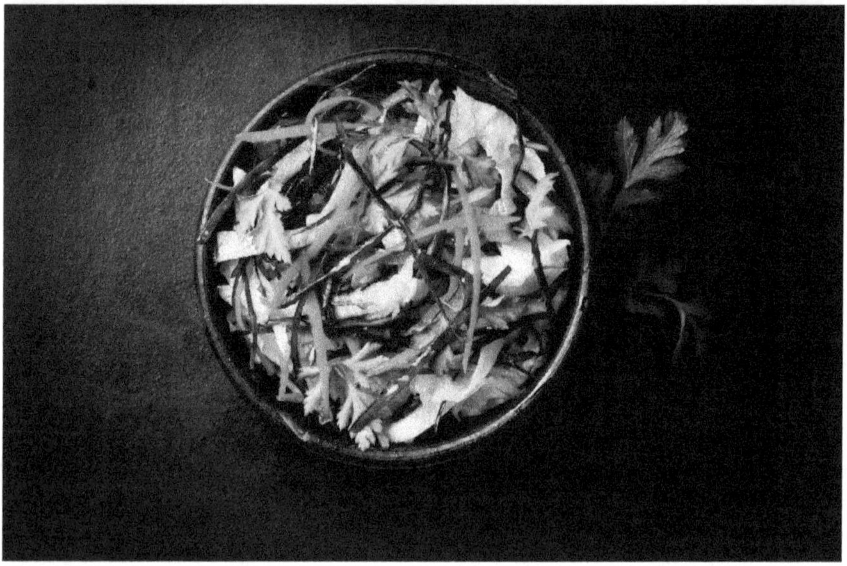

DINNER

14. Corn and Potato Chowder

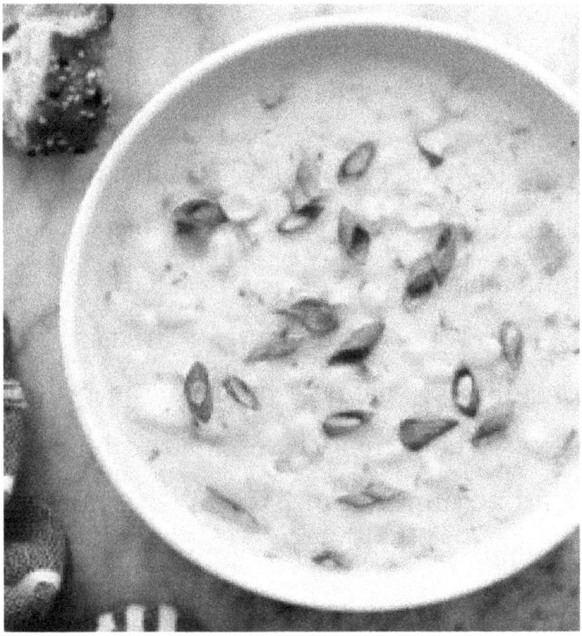

Preparation time: 5 minutes

Cooking time: 35 minutes

Servings: 4

Ingredients:

- 2 ears of corn
- 10 ounces tofu, extra-firm, drained cubed
- 1 1/2 cups frozen corn kernels
- 1/4 medium onion, peeled, chopped

- 3 medium potatoes, peeled, cubed
- 1/4 medium red bell pepper, cored, chopped
- ¼ cup cilantro, chopped
- 2/3 teaspoon salt
- 1/4 cup coconut cream
- 7 cups of vegetable broth

Directions:

1. Prepare the ears of corn and for this, remove their skin and husk, then cut each corn into four pieces and place them in a large pot.
2. Place the pot over medium-high heat, add cilantro, onion and bell pepper, pour in the broth, bring the mixture to boil, then switch heat to medium level and cook for 20 minutes until corn pieces are tender.
3. Add potatoes, cook for 8 minutes until fork tender, then add tofu and kernels, simmer for 5 minutes and taste to adjust seasoning.
4. Remove pot from heat, stir in cream until combined and serve straight away.

Nutrition: Calories: 159 Fat: 2.4 g Carbs: 29 g Protein: 6.6 g

15. Cauliflower Soup

Preparation time: 10 minutes

Cooking time: 40 minutes

Servings: 2

Ingredients:

- 1 small head of cauliflower, slice into florets
- 4 tablespoons pomegranate seeds
- 2 sprigs of thyme and more for garnishing
- 1 teaspoon minced garlic
- 2/3 teaspoon salt
- 1/3 teaspoon ground black pepper
- 1 tablespoon olive oil
- 1 1/2 cups vegetable stock
- 1/2 cup coconut milk, unsweetened

Directions:

1. Take a pot, place it over medium heat, add oil and when hot, add garlic and cook for 1 minute until fragrant. Add florets, thyme, pour in the stock and bring the mixture to boil.
2. Switch heat to the medium low level, simmer the soup for 30 minutes until florets are tender, then remove the pot from heat, discard the thyme and puree using an immersion blender until smooth.

3. Stir milk into the soup, season with salt and black pepper, then garnish with pomegranate seeds and thyme sprigs and serve.

Nutrition: Calories: 184 Fat: 11 g Carbs: 17 g Protein: 3 g

16. Red Pepper and Tomato Soup

Preparation time: 10 minutes

Cooking time: 40 minutes

Servings: 4

Ingredients:

- 2 carrots, peeled, chopped
- 1 1/4 pounds red bell peppers, deseeded, sliced into quarters
- 1/2 of medium red onion, peeled, sliced into thin wedges
- 16 ounces small tomatoes, halved
- 1 tablespoon chopped basil
- 1/2 teaspoon salt
- 2 cups vegetable broth

Directions:

1. Switch on the oven, then set it to 450 F and let it preheat. Then place all the vegetables in a single on a baking sheet lined with foil and roast for 40 minutes until the skins of peppers are slightly charred.
2. When done, remove the baking sheet from the oven, let them cool for 10 minutes, then peel the peppers and transfer all the vegetables into a blender.

3. Add basil and salt to the vegetables, pour in the broth, and puree the vegetables until smooth. Serve straight away.

Nutrition: Calories: 77.4 Fat: 1.8 g Carbs: 14.4 g Protein: 3.3 g

17. Wonton Soup

Preparation time: 15 minutes

Cooking time: 10 minutes

Servings: 4

Ingredients:

For the Soup:

- 4 cups vegetable broth
- 2 green onions, chopped

For the Wontons Filling:

- 1 cup chopped mushrooms
- 1/4 cup walnuts, chopped
- 1 green onion, chopped
- 1/2 inch of ginger, grated
- ½ teaspoon minced garlic
- 1 tablespoon rice vinegar
- 2 teaspoons soy sauce
- 1 teaspoon brown sugar
- 20 Vegan Wonton Wrappers

Directions:

1. Prepare wonton filling and for this, take a bowl, place all the ingredients in it, except for wrapper and toss until well combined.

2. Place a wonton wrapper on working space, place 1 teaspoon of prepared filling in the middle, then brush some water at the edges, fold over to shape like a half-moon, and seal the wrappers by pinching the edges.
3. Take a large pot, place it over medium-high heat, add broth, and bring it to boil. Then drop prepared wontons in it, one at a time, and boil for 5 minutes. When cooked, garnish the soup with green onions and serve.

Nutrition: Calories: 196.9 Fat: 4 g Carbs: 31 g Protein: 6.6 g

18. Spicy Cilantro and Coconut Soup

Preparation time: 15 minutes

Cooking time: 3-5 minutes

Servings: 2

Ingredients:

- 2 tbsp cilantro leaves
- jalapeno
- 1 tbsp lime juice
- 13 ½ oz full-fat coconut milk
- ¼ tsp sea salt
- 3 cloves crushed garlic
- ¼ cup diced onion
- 2 tbsp avocado oil

Directions:

1. Add the avocado oil to a medium pan and heat. Add in the salt, garlic, and onion, cooking for 3 to 5 minutes, either that or till the onion bulbs get to be smooth.
2. Put in the onion mixture, cilantro, jalapeno, lime juice, and coconut milk to a blender and mix until it becomes creamy. Pour into a bowl and enjoy.

Nutrition: Calories: 114 Carbs: 14g Fat: 5g Protein: 2g

19. Tarragon Soup

Preparation time: 15 minutes

Cooking time: 0 minutes

Servings: 2

Ingredients:

- 2 tbsp chopped fresh tarragon
- celery stalk
- ½ cup raw cashews
- 1 tbsp lemon juice
- 13 ½ oz full-fat coconut milk
- ½ tsp pepper, divided
- ½ tsp sea salt, divided
- 3 cloves crushed garlic
- ½ cup diced onion
- 1 tbsp avocado oil

Directions:

1. Add the oil to a medium pan and warm it up. Put in all the seasonings: pepper, salt, garlic bulbs, together with onion bulbs then prepare approximately three to five minutes, or until the onions turn soft.
2. Using a high-speed blender, add the onion mixture, tarragon, celery, cashews, lemon juice, and coconut

milk. Blend everything together until smooth. Taste and adjust the seasonings as you need to.

3. Divide into two bowls and enjoy. You can also add back into a pot and heat through before serving.

Nutrition: Calories: 250 Carbs: 21g Fat: 15g Protein: 6g

20. Asparagus and Artichoke Soup

Preparation time: 15 minutes

Cooking time: 20 minutes

Servings: 4

Ingredients:

- 1 can stemmed and halved artichoke hearts
- 2 cups almond milk
- ½ tsp pepper
- 1/2 tsp sea salt
- 2 cups vegetable broth
- 8 stalks diced asparagus
- 1 cup cubed potatoes
- 2 cloves crushed garlic
- 1 tbsp avocado oil
- ½ cup diced onion

Directions:

1. Add the garlic, avocado oil, and onion in a skillet and cook for a few minutes, either that or till the onion bulbs have smoothened and weakened.
2. Put in the cooked veggies to a pot and add in the pepper, salt, vegetable broth, asparagus, and potatoes. Stir everything together and let it come up to a simmer.

3. Lower the hot temperature and boil gently on about 18 up to 20 minutes, or till the potatoes have become soft.
4. Add in some extra broth if you find that you need to so that the liquid stays about an inch over the veggies. Set the pot away from the fire then let it chill.
5. Using a blender, mix up the cooled soup with the artichokes and almond milk until everything is well-combined and smooth.
6. Adjust any of the seasonings that you need to. You can add extra broth or milk to thick it out if needed. Pour back into the pot and let it warm over low until ready to serve.

Nutrition: Calories: 436 Carbs: 37g Fat: 24g Protein: 18g

SNACKS

21. Vegan Eggplant Patties

Preparation time: 30 minutes

Cooking time: 15 minutes

Servings: 6

Ingredients

- 2 big eggplants
- 1 onion finely diced
- 1 tbsp smashed garlic cloves
- 1 bunch raw parsley, chopped
- 1/2 cup almond meal
- 4 tbsp kalamata olives, pitted and sliced
- 1 tbsp baking soda
- salt and ground pepper to taste
- olive oil or avocado oil, for frying

Directions

1. Peel off eggplants, rinse, and cut in half. Sauté eggplant cubes in a non-stick skillet - occasionally stirring - about 10 minutes.

2. Transfer to a large bowl and mash with an immersion blender. Add eggplant puree into a bowl and add in all remaining ingredients (except oil).
3. Knead a mixture using your hands until the dough is smooth, sticky, and easy to shape. Shape mixture into 6 patties.
4. Heat-up the olive oil in a frying skillet on medium-high heat. Fry patties for about 3 to 4 minutes per side. Remove patties on a platter lined with kitchen paper towel to drain. Serve warm.

Nutrition: Calories: 210 Carbs: 16g Fat: 12g Protein: 8g

22. Spinach Chips

Preparation time: 10 minutes

Cooking time: 20 minutes

Servings: 4

Ingredients:

- 1 pound baby spinach, well dried
- Salt and black pepper to the taste
- ½ teaspoon oregano, dried
- 1 teaspoon sweet paprika
- Cooking spray

Directions:

1. Oiled a baking sheet using cooking spray and spread the spinach leaves on it. Add the other ingredients, toss gently and bake at 435 degrees F for 20 minutes. Serve as a snack.

Nutrition: Calories 140 Fat 4.2g Carbs 6g Protein 4g

23. Balsamic Zucchini Bowls

Preparation time: 10 minutes

Cooking time: 3 hours

Servings: 8

Ingredients:

- 3 zucchinis, thinly sliced
- Salt and black pepper to the taste
- 2 tablespoons olive oil
- 1 teaspoon turmeric powder
- 1 teaspoon coriander, ground
- 2 tablespoons balsamic vinegar

Directions:

1. Spread the zucchini on a lined baking sheet and mix with the other ingredients. Toss and bake at 360 degrees F for 3 hours. Divide into bowls and serve as a snack.

Nutrition: Calories 100 Fat 3g Carbs 3g Protein 4.5g

24. Spinach Spread

Preparation time: 10 minutes

Cooking time: 0 minutes

Servings: 5

Ingredients:

- 4 cups spinach, chopped
- ¼ cup olive oil
- Salt and black pepper to the taste
- 4 garlic cloves, minced
- ¾ cup tahini
- ½ cup lime juice
- Zest of 1 lime, grated
- 1 tablespoon oregano, chopped
- 1 tablespoon chives, chopped

Directions:

1. In your blender, mix the spinach with the oil and the other ingredients, pulse well and serve as a party spread.

Nutrition: Calories 110 Fat 5.1g Carbs 6.2g Protein 3.3g

25. Kale Spread

Preparation time: 10 minutes

Cooking time: 0 minutes

Servings: 2

Ingredients:

- 3 cups kale, chopped
- 3 tablespoons tomato sauce
- ¼ cup avocado mayonnaise
- Salt and black pepper to the taste
- 1 teaspoon mint, chopped
- 1 teaspoon turmeric powder
- ½ teaspoon garlic powder

Directions:

1. In a blender, mix the kale with the tomato sauce and the other ingredients, blend well and serve.

Nutrition: Calories 100 Fat 12g Carbs 1g Protein 6g

VEGETABLES

26. Pinto and Green Bean Fry with Couscous

Preparation Time: 5 Minutes

Cooking Time: 15 Minutes

Serving: 4

Ingredients:

- 1/2 cup water
- 1/3 cup couscous (semolina or whole-wheat)
- 2 tablespoons extra-virgin olive oil
- 1 small onion, chopped
- 1/2 tablespoon minced garlic
- 1 cup green beans, cut into 1-inch pieces
- 1 cup fresh or frozen corn
- 11/2 teaspoons chili powder
- 1/2 teaspoon ground cumin
- 1 large tomato, finely chopped
- 1 (14-ounce) can pinto beans, drained and rinsed
- 1 teaspoon salt

Directions:

1. Bring the water to a boil in a small saucepan. Remove from the heat and stir in the couscous. Cover the pan and let sit for 10 minutes.
2. Gently fluff the couscous with a fork.
3. While the couscous is cooking, heat the olive oil in a large skillet over medium heat. Add the onion and garlic and stir for 1 minute.
4. Add the green beans and stir for 4 minutes, until they begin to soften.
5. Add the corn, stir for another 2 minutes, then add the chili powder and cumin, and stir to coat the vegetables.
6. Add the tomato and simmer for 3 or 4 minutes. Stir in the pinto beans and couscous and cook for 3 to 4 minutes, until everything is heated throughout. Stir often.
7. Stir in the salt and serve hot or warm.

Nutrition: Calories: 267Total Fat: 8gTotal Carbs: 41g Fiber: 10g Sugar: 4 g Protein: 10g Sodium: 601mg

27. Indonesian-Style Spicy Fried Tempeh Strips

Preparation Time: 5 Minutes

Cooking Time: 20 Minutes

Serving: 4

Ingredients:

- 1 cup sesame oil, or as needed
- 1 (12-ounce) package tempeh, cut into narrow 2-inch strips
- 2 medium onions, sliced
- 11/2 tablespoons tomato paste
- 3 teaspoons tamari or soy sauce
- 1 teaspoon dried red chili flakes
- 1/2 teaspoon brown sugar
- 2 tablespoons lime juice

Directions:

1. Heat the sesame oil in a large wok or saucepan over medium-high heat. Add more sesame oil as needed to raise the level to at least 1 inch.

2. As soon as the oil is hot but not smoking, add the tempeh slices and cook, stirring frequently, for 10 minutes, until a light golden color on all sides.
3. Add the onions and stir for another 10 minutes, until the tempeh and onions are brown and crispy.
4. Remove with a slotted spoon and add to a large bowl lined with several sheets of paper towel.
5. While the tempeh and onions are cooking, whisk together the tomato paste, tamari or soy sauce, red chili flakes, brown sugar, and lime juice in a small bowl.
6. Remove the paper towel from the large bowl and pour the sauce over the tempeh strips. Mix well to coat.

Nutrition: Calories: 317 Total Fat: 23g Total Carbs: 15g Sugar: 4g Protein: 17gSodium: 266mg

SALAD

28. Cucumber Tomato Chopped Salad

Preparation Time: 15 minutes

Cooking Time: 0 minute

Servings: 6

Ingredients:

- ½ cup light mayonnaise
- 1 tablespoon lemon juice
- 1 tablespoon fresh dill, chopped
- 1 tablespoon chives, chopped
- ½ cup feta cheese, crumbled
- Salt and pepper to taste
- 1 red onion, chopped
- 1 cucumber, diced
- 1 radish, diced
- 3 tomatoes, diced
- Chives, chopped

Directions:

1. Combine the mayo, lemon juice, fresh dill, chives, feta cheese, salt and pepper in a bowl.
2. Mix well.

3. Stir in the onion, cucumber, radish and tomatoes.
4. Coat evenly.
5. Garnish with the chopped chives.

Nutrition: Calories 187 Fat 16.7 g Saturated fat 4.1 g Carbohydrates 6.7 g Fiber 2 g Protein 3.3 g

29. Zucchini Pasta Salad

Preparation Time: 4 minutes

Cooking Time: 0 minute

Servings: 15

Ingredients:

- 5 tablespoons olive oil
- 2 teaspoons Dijon mustard
- 3 tablespoons red-wine vinegar
- 1 clove garlic, grated
- 2 tablespoons fresh oregano, chopped
- 1 shallot, chopped
- ¼ teaspoon red pepper flakes
- 16 oz. zucchini noodles
- ¼ cup Kalamata olives, pitted
- 3 cups cherry tomatoes, sliced in half
- ¾ cup Parmesan cheese, shaved

Instructions:

1. Mix the olive oil, Dijon mustard, red-wine vinegar, garlic, oregano, shallot and red pepper flakes in a bowl.
2. Stir in the zucchini noodles.

3. Sprinkle on top the olives, tomatoes and Parmesan cheese.

Nutrition: Calories 299 Fat 24.7 g Saturated fat 5.1 g Carbohydrates 11.6 g Fiber 2.8 g Protein 7 g

GRAINS

30. Raw Noodles with Avocado 'N Nuts

Preparation Time: 5 minutes

Cooking Time: 10 minutes

Servings: 2

Ingredients:

- 1 zucchini
- 1½ c. basil
- 1/3 c. water
- 5 tbsps. pine nuts
- 2 tbsps. lemon juice
- 1 avocado, peeled, pitted, sliced
- Optional: 2 tbsps. olive oil
- 6 yellow cherry tomatoes, halved
- Optional: 6 red cherry tomatoes, halved
- Sea salt and black pepper

Directions:

1. Add the basil, water, nuts, lemon juice, avocado slices, optional olive oil (if desired), salt, and pepper to a blender.

2. Blend the ingredients into a smooth mixture. Season with more pepper and salt and blend again.
3. Divide the sauce and the zucchini noodles between two medium-sized bowls for serving, and combine in each.
4. Top the mixtures with the halved yellow cherry tomatoes, and the optional red cherry tomatoes (if desired);

Nutrition: Calories 317, Carbs 7.4 g, Fats 28.1 g, Protein 7.2 g

31. Rice & Bean Burritos

Preparation Time: 10 minutes

Cooking Time: 15 minutes

Servings: 8

Ingredients:

- 32 oz. fat-free refried beans
- 6 tortillas
- 2 c. cooked rice
- ½ c. salsa
- 1 tbsp. olive oil
- 1 bunch green onions, chopped
- 2 bell peppers, chopped
- Guacamole

Directions:

1. Preheat the oven to 375°F.
2. Dump the refried beans into a saucepan and place over medium heat to warm.
3. Heat the tortillas and lay them out on a flat surface.
4. Spoon the beans in a long mound that runs across the tortilla, just a little off from center.
5. Spoon some rice and salsa over the beans; add the green pepper and onions to taste, along with any other finely chopped vegetables you like.

6. Fold over the shortest edge of the plain tortilla and roll it up, folding in the sides as you go.
7. Place each burrito, seam side down, on a nonstick-sprayed baking sheet.
8. Brush with olive oil and bake for 15 minutes.

Nutrition: Calories 290, Carbs 49 g, Fats 6 g, Protein 9 g

LEGUMES

32. Old-Fashioned Lentil and Vegetable Stew

Preparation Time: 10 minutes

Cooking Time: 10 minutes

Servings: 4

Ingredients:

- 3 tablespoons olive oil
- 1 large onion, chopped
- 1 carrot, chopped
- 1 bell pepper, diced
- 1 habanero pepper, chopped
- 3 cloves garlic, minced
- Kosher salt and black pepper, to taste
- 1 teaspoon ground cumin
- 1 teaspoon smoked paprika
- 1 (28-ounce) can tomatoes, crushed
- 2 tablespoons tomato ketchup
- 4 cups vegetable broth

- 3/4-pound dry red lentils, soaked overnight and drained
- 1 avocado, sliced

Directions

1. In a heavy-bottomed pot, heat the olive oil over medium heat. Once hot, sauté the onion, carrot and peppers for about 4 minutes.
2. Sauté the garlic for about 1 minute or so.
3. Add in the spices, tomatoes, ketchup, broth and canned lentils. Let it simmer, stirring occasionally, for about 20 minutes or until cooked through.
4. Serve garnished with the slices of avocado. Bon appétit!

Nutrition: Calories: 475; Fat: 17.3g; Carbs: 61.4g; Protein: 23.7g

BREAD & PIZZA

33. Moist Banana Bread

Preparation Time: 10 Minutes

Cooking Time: 60 Minutes

Servings: 6

Ingredients:

- Eggs – 2
- Baking powder – 1 teaspoon.
- Sugar – 1/2 cup
- Vanilla – 1 teaspoon.
- Butter – 1/2 cup, melted
- Ripe bananas – 3
- All-purpose flour – 1 1/2 cups
- Pinch of salt

Directions:

1. Preheat the oven to 350 F. In a large bowl, add bananas and mash until smooth. Add eggs, vanilla, butter, and mix well.
2. Add flour, baking powder, sugar, and salt and mix until well combined.

3. Pour batter into the greased loaf pan and bake in a preheated oven for 60 minutes. Slice and serve.

Nutrition: Calories 388, Carbs 54.6g, Fat 17.3g, Protein 5.9g

SOUP AND STEW

34. Garden Vegetable and Herb Soup

Preparation Time: 20 minutes

Cooking Time: 30 minutes

Servings: 8

Ingredients:

- 2 tablespoons olive oil
- 2 medium onions, hacked
- 2 huge carrots, cut
- 1-pound red potatoes (around 3 medium), cubed
- 2 cups of water
- 1 can (14-1/2 ounces) diced tomatoes in sauce
- 1-1/2 cups vegetable soup
- 1-1/2 teaspoons garlic powder
- 1 teaspoon dried basil
- 1/2 teaspoon salt
- 1/2 teaspoon paprika
- 1/4 teaspoon dill weed
- 1/4 teaspoon pepper
- 1 medium yellow summer squash, split and cut
- 1 medium zucchini, split and cut

Directions:

1. In a huge pan, heat oil over medium warmth. Include onions and carrots; cook and mix until onions are delicate, 4-6 minutes. Include potatoes and cook 2 minutes. Mix in water, tomatoes, juices, and seasonings.
2. Heat to the point of boiling. Diminish heat; stew, revealed, until potatoes and carrots are delicate, 9 minutes.
3. Include yellow squash and zucchini; cook until vegetables are delicate, 9 minutes longer. Serve or, whenever wanted, puree blend in clusters, including extra stock until desired consistency is accomplished.

Nutrition: kcal: 252 Carbohydrates: 12 g Protein: 1 g Fat: 11 g

35. The Mediterranean Delight with Fresh Vinaigrette

Preparation Time: 5 minutes

Cooking Time: 10 minutes

Servings: 2

Ingredients:

- Herbed citrus vinaigrette:
- 1 tablespoon of lemon juice
- 2 tablespoons of orange juice
- ½ teaspoon of lemon zest
- ½ teaspoon of orange zest
- 2 tablespoons of olive oil
- 1 tablespoon of finely chopped fresh oregano leaves
- Salt to taste
- Black pepper to taste
- 2-3 tablespoons of freshly julienned mint leaves
- Salad:
- 1 freshly diced medium-sized cucumber
- 2 cups of cooked and rinsed chickpeas
- ½ cup of freshly diced red onion
- 2 freshly diced medium-sized tomatoes
- 1 freshly diced red bell pepper

- ¼ cup of green olives
- ½ cup of pomegranates

Directions:

1. In a large salad bowl, add the juice and zest of both the lemon and the orange and oregano and olive oil. Whisk together so that they are mixed well. Season the vinaigrette with salt and pepper to taste.
2. After draining the chickpeas, add them to the dressing. Then, add the onions. Give them a thorough mix, so that the onion and chickpeas absorb the flavors.
3. Now, chop the rest of the veggies and start adding them to the salad bowl. Give them a good toss.
4. Lastly, add the olives and fresh mint. Adjust the salt and pepper as required.
5. Serve this Mediterranean delight chilled – a cool summer salad that is good for the tummy and the soul.

Nutrition: kcal: 286 Carbohydrates: 29 g Protein: 1 g Fat: 11 g

SAUCE, DRESSINGS & DIP

36. Lemon Tahini

Preparation time: 15 minutes

Cooking time: 0 minutes

Servings: 4

Ingredients:

- 1/4 cup fresh lemon juice
- 4 medium garlic cloves, pressed
- 1/2 cup tahini
- 1/2 teaspoon fine sea salt
- Pinch of ground cumin
- 6 tablespoons ice water

Directions:

1. In a medium bowl, combine the lemon juice and garlic and set aside for 10 minutes.
2. Through a fine-mesh sieve, strain the mixture into another medium bowl, pressing the garlic solids.
3. Discard the garlic solids.
4. In the lemon juice bowl, add the tahini, salt, and cumin, and whisk until well blended.

5. Slowly, add water, 2 tablespoons at a time, whisking well after each addition.

Nutrition: Calories 187 Total Fat 16.3 g Saturated Fat 2.4 g Cholesterol 0 mgSodium 273 mg Total Carbs 7.7 gFiber 2.9 g Sugar 0.5 g Protein 5.4 g

37. Keto-Vegan Ketchup

Preparation time: 35 minutes

Cooking time: 11 minutes

Servings: 12

Ingredients:

- 1/8 t of the following:
- Mustard powder
- Cloves, ground
- 1/4 t. paprika
- 1/2 t. garlic powder
- 3/4 t. onion powder
- 1 t. sea salt
- 3 tablespoons. apple cider vinegar
- 1/4 c. powdered monk fruit
- 1 c. water
- 6 oz. tomato paste

Directions:

1. In a little saucepan, whisk together all the **Ingredients:**
2. Cover the pan and bring to low heat and simmer for 30 minutes, stirring occasionally.

3. Once reduced, add to the blender and puree until it's a smooth consistency.

Nutrition: Calories: 13 Carbohydrates: 2 g Proteins: 0 g Fats: 0 g

38. Italian Stuffed Artichokes

Preparation Time: 20 minutes

Cooking Time: 25 minutes

Servings: 4

Ingredients:

- 4 large artichokes
- 2 teaspoon lemon juice
- 2 cups soft Italian bread crumbs, toasted
- 1/2 cup grated Parmigiano-Reggiano cheese
- 1/2 cup minced fresh parsley
- 2 teaspoon Italian seasoning
- 1 teaspoon grated lemon peel
- 1/2 teaspoon pepper
- 1/4 teaspoon salt
- 1 tablespoon olive oil

Directions:

1. Level the bottom of each artichoke using a sharp knife and trim off 1-inch from the tops. Snip off tips of outer leaves using kitchen scissors, then brush lemon juice on cut edges. In a Dutch oven, stand the artichokes and pour 1-inch of water, then boil. Lower the heat, put the cover, and let it simmer for 5 minutes or until the leaves near the middle pull out effortlessly.

2. Turn the artichokes upside down to drain. Allow it to stand for 10 minutes. Carefully scrape out the fuzzy middle part of the artichokes using a spoon and get rid of it.
3. Mix the salt, pepper, lemon peel, Italian seasoning, garlic, parsley, cheese, and breadcrumbs in a small bowl, then add olive oil and stir well. Gently spread the artichoke leaves apart, then fill it with breadcrumb mixture.
4. Put it in a cooking spray-coated 11x7-inch baking dish. Let it bake for 10 minutes at 350 degrees F without cover, or until the filling turns light brown.

Nutrition: calories 543 fat 5 carbs 44 protein 6

APPETIZER

39. Cookie in A Mug

Preparation time: 5 minutes

Cooking time: 2 minutes

Servings: 1

Ingredients:

- 1 egg yolk
- 1 pinch cinnamon
- 1 pinch salt
- 1 tbsp butter
- 1 tbsp erythritol
- 1/8 tsp vanilla extract
- 2 tbsp sugar free chocolate chips
- 3 tbsp almond flour

Directions:

1. In a microwave safe mug or ramekin, melt butter in microwave. Stir in cinnamon, salt, erythritol, and vanilla. Mix well. Add egg yolk and mix well.

2. Stir in almond flour. Mix well. Fold in chocolate chips. Press on bottom of mug or ramekin. On high, cook in microwave for a minute and 10 seconds. Serve and enjoy.

Nutrition: Calories: 330Protein: 7.0gCarbs: 4.0gFat: 31.0g

40. Fudgy Choco-Peanut Butter

Preparation time: 15 minutes

Cooking time: 0 minutes

Servings: 32

Ingredients:

- 4 ounces cream cheese (softened)
- 2 tablespoons unsweetened cocoa powder
- 1/2 cup butter
- 1/2 cup natural peanut butter
- 1/2 teaspoon vanilla extract
- 1/4 cup powdered erythritol

Directions:

1. In microwave safe bowl, mix peanut butter and butter. Microwave for 10-second interval until melted. While mixing every after sticking in the microwave.
2. Mix in vanilla extract, cocoa powder, erythritol, and cream cheese. Thoroughly mix. Line an 8x8-inch baking pan with foil and evenly spread mixture.
3. Place in the fridge to set and slice into 32 equal squares.
4. Store in tightly lidded container in the fridge and enjoy as a snack.

Nutrition: Calories: 65 Protein: 1.5g Carbs: 1.0g Fat: 6.0g

41. Vegan Fudgy Granola Bar

Preparation time: 15 minutes

Cooking time: 25 minutes

Servings: 16

Ingredients:

- 1 pinch salt
- 1 1/2 cups sliced almonds
- 1/2 cup flaked coconut (unsweetened)
- 1/2 cup pecans
- 1/2 cup sunflower seeds
- 1/2 cup dried, unsweetened cranberries (chopped)
- 1/2 cup butter
- 1/2 cup powdered erythritol
- 1/2 tsp vanilla extract

Directions:

1. With parchment paper line a square baking dish and preheat oven to 300F. In food processor, pulse sunflower seeds, pecans, coconut, and almonds until crumb like.
2. In a bowl, add pinch of salt and cranberries. Stir in crumb mixture and mix well. In microwave safe mug, melt butter in 20-second interval. Whisk in vanilla

extract and erythritol. Pour over granola crumbs and mix well.

3. Press mixture as compact as you can on prepared dish. Pop in the oven and bake for 25 minutes. Let it cool and cut into 16 equal squares.

Nutrition: Calories: 180Protein: 4.0gCarbs: 5.0gFat: 17.0g

SMOOTHIES AND JUICES

42. Classic Switchel

Preparation Time: 5 minutes

Cooking Time: 0 minutes

Servings: 4

Ingredients:

- 1-inch piece ginger, minced
- 2 tablespoons apple cider vinegar
- 2 tablespoons maple syrup
- 4 cups water
- ¼ teaspoon sea salt, optional

Directions:

1. Combine all the ingredients in a glass. Stir to mix well.
2. Serve immediately or chill in the refrigerator for an hour before serving.

Nutrition: calories: 110fat: 0gcarbs: 28.0gfiber: 0gprotein: 0g

43. Lime and Cucumber Electrolyte Drink

Preparation Time: 5 minutes

Cooking Time: 0 minutes

Servings: 4

Ingredients:

- ¼ cup chopped cucumber
- 1 tablespoon fresh lime juice
- 1 tablespoon apple cider vinegar
- 2 tablespoons maple syrup
- ¼ teaspoon sea salt, optional
- 4 cups water

Directions:

1. Combine all the ingredients in a glass. Stir to mix well.
2. Refrigerate overnight before serving.

Nutrition: calories: 114fat: 0.1gcarbs: 28.9gfiber: 0.3gprotein: 0.3g

DESSERTS

44. Cherry-Vanilla Rice Pudding

Preparation time: 15 minutes

Cooking time: 30 minutes

Servings: 4-6

Ingredients:

- 1 cup short-grain brown rice
- 1¾ cups nondairy milk, plus more as needed
- 1½ cups water
- 4 tablespoons unrefined sugar or pure maple syrup (use 2 tablespoons if you use a sweetened milk), plus more as needed
- 1 teaspoon vanilla extract (use ½ teaspoon if you use vanilla milk)
- Pinch salt
- ¼ cup dried cherries or ½ cup fresh or frozen pitted cherries

Directions:

1. In your electric pressure cooker's cooking pot, combine the rice, milk, water, sugar, vanilla, and salt. High pressure for 30 minutes. Select High Pressure for 30 minutes.
2. Let the pressure release naturally, within 20 minutes. Unlock and remove the lid.
3. Stir in the cherries and put the lid back on loosely for about 10 minutes. Serve, adding more milk or sugar, as desired.

Nutrition: Calories: 177Fat: 1gProtein: 3gCarbs: 2g

45. Lime in The Coconut Chia Pudding

Preparation time: 30 minutes

Cooking time: 0 minutes

Servings: 4

Ingredients:

- Zest and juice of 1 lime
- 1 (14-ounce) can coconut milk
- 1 to 2 dates, or 1 tablespoon coconut or other unrefined sugar, or 1 tablespoon maple syrup, or 10 to 15 drops pure liquid stevia
- 2 tablespoons chia seeds, whole or ground
- 2 teaspoons matcha green tea powder (optional)

Directions:

1. Blend all the ingredients in a blender until smooth. Chill in the fridge within 20 minutes, then serve topped with one or more of the topping ideas.
2. Try blueberries, blackberries, sliced strawberries, Coconut Whipped Cream, or toasted unsweetened coconut.

Nutrition: Calories: 226Fat: 20gCarbs: 13gProtein: 3g

46. Mint Chocolate Chip Sorbet

Preparation time: 5 minutes

Cooking time: 0 minutes

Servings: 1

Ingredients:

- 1 frozen banana
- 1 tablespoon almond butter/peanut butter, or other nut or seed butter
- 2 tablespoons fresh mint, minced
- ¼ cup or less non-dairy milk (only if needed)
- 2 to 3 tablespoons non-dairy chocolate chips, or cocoa nibs
- 2 to 3 tablespoons goji berries (optional)

Directions:

1. Put the banana, almond butter, and mint in a food processor or blender and purée until smooth.
2. Add the non-dairy milk if needed to keep blending (but only if needed, as this will make the texture less solid).
3. Pulse the chocolate chips and goji berries (if using) into the mix so they're roughly chopped up.

Nutrition: Calories: 212Fat: 10gCarbs: 31gProtein: 3g

47. Peach-Mango Crumble

Preparation time: 15 minutes

Cooking time: 6 minutes

Servings: 4-6

Ingredients:

- 3 cups chopped fresh or frozen peaches
- 3 cups chopped fresh or frozen mangos
- 4 tablespoons unrefined sugar or pure maple syrup, divided
- 1 cup gluten-free rolled oats
- ½ cup shredded coconut, sweetened or unsweetened
- 2 tablespoons coconut oil or vegan margarine

Directions:

1. In a 6- to 7-inch round baking dish, toss together the peaches, mangos, and 2 tablespoons of sugar. In a food processor, combine the oats, coconut, coconut oil, and remaining 2 tablespoons of sugar.
2. Pulse until combined. (If you use maple syrup, you'll need less coconut oil. Start with just the syrup and add oil if the mixture isn't sticking together.) Sprinkle the oat mixture over the fruit mixture.

3. Cover the dish with aluminum foil. Put a trivet in the bottom of your electric pressure cooker's cooking pot and pour in a cup or two of water.
4. Using a foil sling or silicone helper handles, lower the pan onto the trivet. High pressure for 6 minutes.
5. Select High Pressure for 6 minutes; then quick release the pressure. Unlock and remove the lid.
6. Let cool for a few minutes before carefully lifting out the dish with oven mitts or tongs. Scoop out portions to serve.

Nutrition: Calories: 321Fat: 18gProtein: 4gCarbs: 7g

48. Zesty Orange-Cranberry Energy Bites

Preparation time: 25 minutes

Cooking time: 0 minutes

Servings: 12

Ingredients:

- 2 tablespoons almond butter, or cashew or sunflower seed butter
- 2 tablespoons maple syrup, or brown rice syrup
- ¾ cup cooked quinoa
- ¼ cup sesame seeds, toasted
- 1 tablespoon chia seeds
- ½ teaspoon almond extract, or vanilla extract
- Zest of 1 orange
- 1 tablespoon dried cranberries
- ¼ cup ground almonds

Directions:

1. In a medium bowl, mix together the nut or seed butter and syrup until smooth and creamy. Stir in the rest of the fixings, and mix to make sure the consistency is holding together in a ball. Form the mix into 12 balls.
2. Place them on a baking sheet lined with parchment or waxed paper and put in the fridge to set for about 15 minutes.

3. If your balls aren't holding together, it's likely because of the moisture content of your cooked quinoa. Add more nut or seed butter mixed with syrup until it all sticks together.

Nutrition: Calories: 109Fat: 7gCarbs: 11gProtein: 3g

49. “Frosty” Chocolate Shake

Preparation time: 40 minutes

Cooking time: 0 minutes

Servings: 2

Ingredients:

- 1 cup heavy (whipping) cream/coconut cream
- 2 tablespoons unsweetened cocoa powder
- 1 tablespoon almond butter
- 1 teaspoon vanilla extract
- 5 or 6 drops liquid stevia

Directions:

1. Beat the cream in a medium bowl or using a stand mixer until fluffy, 3 to 4 minutes. Add the cocoa powder, almond butter, vanilla, and stevia.
2. Beat the mixture for an additional 2 to 3 minutes, or until the mixture has the consistency of whipped cream. Place the bowl in the freezer for 25 to 30 minutes before serving.

Nutrition: Calories: 493 Fat: 49g Protein: 5g Carbs: 8g

50. French Vanilla Ice Cream with Hot Fudge

Preparation time: 10 minutes

Cooking time: 0 minutes

Servings: 2

Ingredients:

- 1¼ cups heavy (whipping) cream, divided
- ¼ cup unsweetened almond milk
- ½ cup Swerve sweetener, divided
- 1½ teaspoons vanilla extract, divided
- 2 ounces unsweetened chocolate, chopped

Directions:

1. Put a bread loaf pan in the freezer to chill for about 20 minutes. In a medium bowl, combine ¾ cup of cream, the almond milk, ¼ cup of Swerve, and ½ teaspoon of vanilla.
2. Mix with a handheld electric mixer for 2 minutes, or until the sweetener has dissolved. Pour the ice-cream mixture into the chilled loaf pan.
3. Place the pan in the freezer. Every half hour, remove the pan, scrape down the sides, and whisk the mixture for about 1 minute. It will get thicker and thicker each time you whisk it.

4. While the ice cream is in the freezer, combine the remaining ½ cup of cream, remaining ¼ cup of Swerve, and the chocolate in a double boiler over medium-low heat.
5. Stir just until the chocolate melts, and then remove the mixture from the heat. Stir in the rest of the 1 teaspoon of vanilla.
6. After 3½ to 4 hours, the ice cream will be thick enough to eat. Scrape down the sides for the last time and scoop out to serve. Pour the warm sauce over the ice cream.

Nutrition: Calories: 719 Fat: 71g Protein: 7g Carbs: 13g

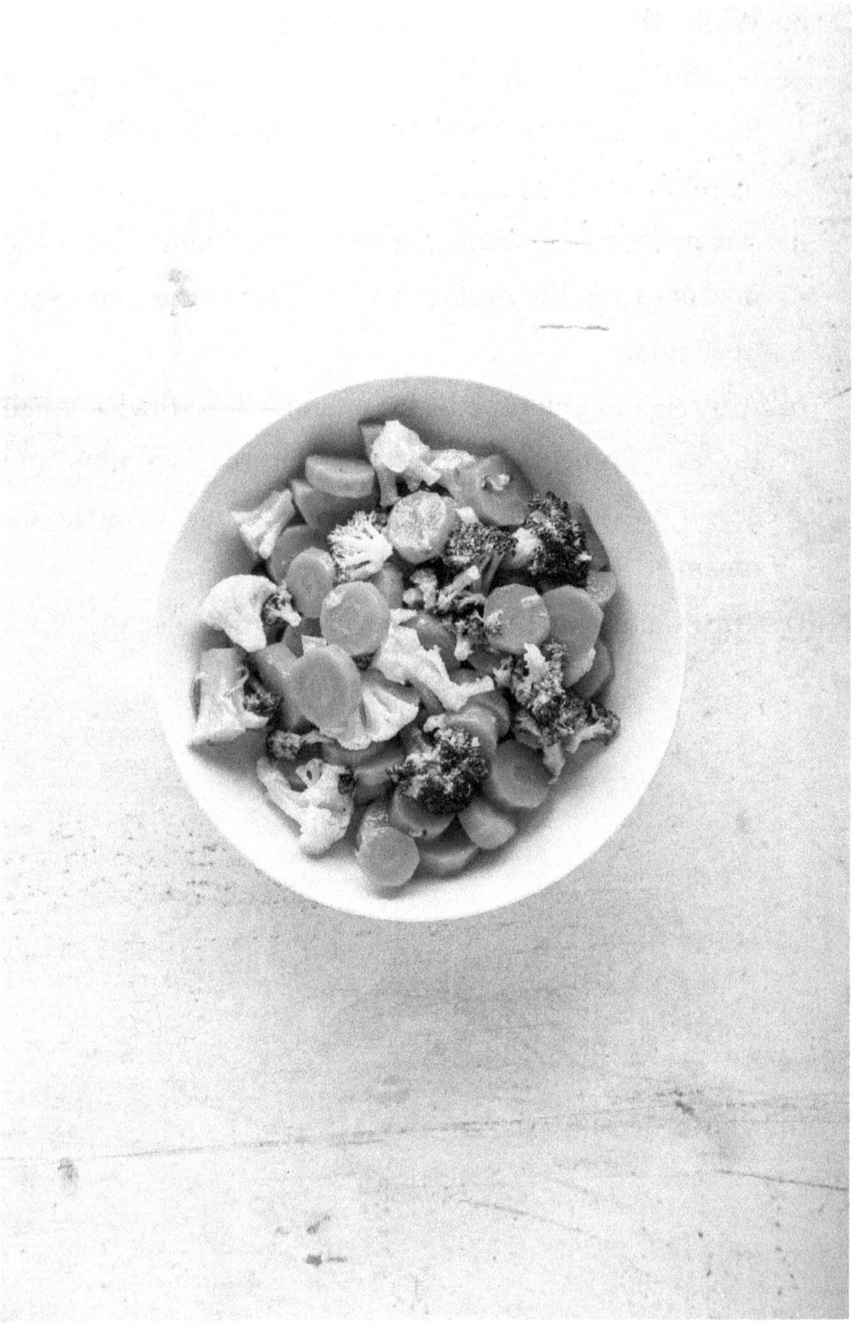

CPSIA information can be obtained
at www.ICGtesting.com
Printed in the USA
BVHW092001220421
605650BV00002B/57

9 781801 832649